WEIGHT LOSS AFTER 40

A Holistic Guide to Thriving in Weight Loss After 40

DR. THOMAS FELAN

Copyright © 2023 by Dr.Thomas Felan

All rights reserved. No part of this publication may be reproduced, distributed, or transmitted in any form or by any means, including photocopying, recording, or other electronic or mechanical methods, without the prior written permission of the publisher, except in the case of brief quotations embodied in critical reviews and certain other noncommercial uses permitted by copyright law.

This book and its contents are protected by copyright. No part of the material protected by this copyright may be reproduced or utilized in any form, electronic or mechanical, including photocopying, recording, or by any information storage and retrieval system, without written permission from the author and publisher.

<u>**DISCLAIMER**</u>

The information provided in this book is for educational and informational purposes only. It is not intended as a substitute for professional medical advice, diagnosis, or treatment. Always seek the advice of your physician or other qualified healthcare provider with any questions you may have regarding a medical condition or treatment.

The content of this book is based on general knowledge and research available up to the time of its publication. Health and medical information are subject to constant advancements and changes. Therefore, the author, publisher, and any contributors to this book make no representations or warranties of any kind, express or implied, regarding the accuracy, completeness, suitability, or applicability of the information contained herein.

Readers are encouraged to consult their healthcare providers before making any changes to their diet, exercise routines, or medical treatment plans. Individual responses to dietary and lifestyle changes can vary, and what works for one person may not work for another.

The author and publisher of this book are not responsible for any adverse effects, injuries, or damages arising from the information provided within these pages. Any reliance you place on the information in this book is strictly at your own risk.

Please consult your healthcare provider before beginning any new dietary or exercise program, making changes to your existing treatment plan, or relying on the information presented in this book. Your healthcare provider is the best source of information regarding your individual health situation.

By reading and utilizing the information in this book, you agree to the terms of this disclaimer. If you do not agree with these terms, please refrain from using this book.

Remember that the field of health and medicine is complex and rapidly evolving. The information in this book is not a substitute for professional medical advice, and readers should always prioritize their health and safety by consulting qualified healthcare professionals.

TABLE OF CONTENT

Introduction

Welcome to the transformative journey of weight loss after 40! Embracing a healthier lifestyle at this stage is not just about shedding pounds; it's a celebration of resilience, wisdom, and the power to redefine your well-being. In this guide, we'll navigate the unique challenges of weight loss after 40, unlocking practical strategies, nutritional insights, and tailored exercises to help you achieve lasting success. Get ready to embark on a path that not only transforms your body but also nurtures a vibrant and fulfilling chapter in your life. Your journey starts now.

Throughout these pages, we'll unravel the intricacies of metabolism changes, explore the role of balanced nutrition, and delve into the nuances of exercise that cater to the needs of your matured body. Hormonal factors, often overlooked, will be demystified, guiding you towards a holistic understanding of your weight management.

But this isn't just about numbers on a scale. It's a holistic approach that embraces the significance of adequate sleep, effective stress management, and the impact of hydration. As we tackle common challenges, you'll find personalized solutions that suit your lifestyle, making the journey enjoyable and sustainable.

Celebrate every small victory, for they are the stepping stones to your success. And when the path seems daunting, consider seeking professional guidance — a support system that can make all the difference.

This guide is more than a manual for weight loss; it's an invitation to reclaim your vitality, rediscover your strength, and embrace the joy of a healthier, more vibrant you. So, let's embark on this empowering journey together!

Understanding Changes in Metabolism

As we venture into the realm of weight loss after 40, understanding the intricate dance of metabolism becomes paramount. Metabolism, the body's engine, undergoes shifts with age, impacting the way we process and store energy. In this section, we'll unravel these changes, shedding light on the factors that may contribute to a slower metabolism.

As we age, muscle mass tends to decline, and since muscles are metabolically active, this can affect the rate at which our bodies burn calories. Additionally, hormonal fluctuations play a crucial role, with shifts in hormones like estrogen and testosterone influencing metabolism and fat distribution.

But fear not, for knowledge is power. By comprehending these metabolic nuances, we gain the tools to navigate them effectively. This section will equip you with insights into optimizing your metabolism through lifestyle choices, nutrition, and targeted exercises, paving the way for a more informed and successful weight loss journey. Let's delve into the science behind metabolism and empower ourselves to make strategic choices for a healthier, more vibrant life.

Discovering the secrets of your metabolism is like deciphering a personalized code that can unlock the doors to effective weight management. We'll explore how strategic meal planning, nutrient-dense foods, and mindful eating can not only support your metabolism but also provide sustained energy throughout the day.

Exercise, another key player, takes center stage as we discuss workouts tailored to boost metabolism and preserve lean muscle mass. It's about finding the right balance, embracing activities that resonate with your body's current needs and capabilities.

So, join me in this exploration of metabolism, where we transform scientific insights into practical strategies. Armed with this knowledge, you'll not only adapt to the changes that come with age but also harness the power of your metabolism to propel you towards your weight loss goals. Get ready to redefine your relationship with your body and metabolism, laying the foundation for a healthier, more vibrant you.

Metabolism, the intricate biochemical process that sustains life, undergoes notable changes as we age, especially after 40. One significant shift is the natural decline in muscle mass, which tends to accompany the aging process. Since muscle tissue is metabolically active, this reduction can lead to a decrease in the number of calories burned at rest, impacting overall metabolic rate.

Furthermore, hormonal fluctuations play a pivotal role. For instance, the decline in estrogen during menopause for women and the gradual decrease in testosterone for men can influence how the body stores and utilizes fat. These hormonal changes may contribute to a redistribution of fat, often resulting in an increase in abdominal fat.

Understanding these metabolic changes is crucial for crafting effective strategies for weight management. It emphasizes the importance of not only adjusting calorie intake but also adopting a holistic approach that includes strength training exercises to preserve and build muscle mass. By appreciating these shifts, you empower yourself to make informed choices, ensuring that your lifestyle aligns with the evolving needs of your body's metabolism. This knowledge forms the cornerstone of a successful and sustainable weight loss journey after 40.

Importance of Balanced Nutrition

In the pursuit of weight loss after 40, the importance of balanced nutrition takes center stage. A well-rounded, nutrient-dense diet isn't just about shedding pounds; it's about providing your body with the essential elements it needs to thrive at every stage of life.

As metabolism experiences changes, the significance of wise nutritional choices becomes even more pronounced. A balanced diet, rich in vitamins, minerals, and macronutrients, not only supports weight management but also promotes overall health. This section will delve into the role of key nutrients, emphasizing the importance of a diverse and colorful plate.

Discover how the right mix of proteins, carbohydrates, fats, vitamins, and minerals can fuel your body, enhance metabolism, and contribute to sustained energy levels.

We'll explore practical tips for meal planning, mindful eating, and making informed choices that align with your weight loss goals and long-term well-being. So, let's embark on a journey to nourish your body from within, embracing the transformative power of balanced nutrition.

Proteins:

- Essential for muscle maintenance and repair.
- Sources include lean meats, poultry, fish, eggs, dairy, legumes, and plant-based options like tofu and tempeh.

Carbohydrates:

- Provide a primary source of energy.
- Opt for complex carbohydrates like whole grains, fruits, vegetables, and legumes for sustained energy and fiber.

Fats:

- Necessary for hormone production and nutrient absorption.
- Choose healthy fats like avocados, nuts, seeds, olive oil, and fatty fish such as salmon.

Vitamins:

- Play a vital role in various bodily functions.
- Include a variety of fruits and vegetables to ensure a broad spectrum of vitamins.

Minerals:

- Essential for bone health, fluid balance, and nerve function.
- Incorporate foods like leafy greens, nuts, seeds, dairy, and whole grains for a diverse mineral intake.

Fiber:

- Supports digestion and helps maintain a feeling of fullness.
- Found in whole grains, fruits, vegetables, legumes, and nuts.

Hydration:

- Often overlooked but crucial for overall health and weight management.

- Water, herbal teas, and infused water with fruits and herbs are excellent choices.

Balanced nutrition involves incorporating these elements in appropriate proportions. It's about creating meals that are not only satisfying but also nourishing, providing your body with the right mix of nutrients for optimal function. As we explore these components, you'll gain insights into crafting a well-balanced diet that supports your weight loss journey while promoting overall health and vitality.

Balancing nutrients in your diet involves creating a harmonious blend of proteins, carbohydrates, fats, vitamins, minerals, and fiber. Here's a guide on how to achieve this nutritional equilibrium:

Portion Control:

- Be mindful of portion sizes to avoid overconsumption of any particular nutrient.
- Use smaller plates to help control portions and prevent overeating.

Diverse Food Choices:

- Incorporate a variety of foods from different food groups to ensure a broad spectrum of nutrients.
- Experiment with different fruits, vegetables, whole grains, lean proteins, and healthy fats.

Protein Distribution:

- Spread protein intake throughout the day to support muscle maintenance and repair.
- Include sources like lean meats, plant-based proteins, and dairy in each meal.

Colorful Plate:

- Aim for a colorful plate with a variety of fruits and vegetables.
- Different colors often indicate diverse nutrient profiles, ensuring you get a range of vitamins and minerals.

Whole Grains:

- Choose whole grains over refined grains for increased fiber and nutrient content.
- Examples include brown rice, quinoa, whole wheat, and oats.

Healthy Fats:

- Incorporate sources of healthy fats, such as avocados, nuts, and olive oil, in moderation.
- These fats contribute to satiety and support various bodily functions.

Hydration:

- Ensure adequate water intake throughout the day.
- Limit sugary drinks and choose water, herbal teas, or infused water options.

Meal Planning:

- Plan meals in advance to ensure a balanced combination of nutrients.
- Consider consulting with a nutritionist for personalized guidance.

Balancing nutrients is about creating a sustainable and enjoyable eating pattern that meets your body's needs. By paying attention to variety, portion sizes, and the quality of your food choices, you can foster a balanced diet that supports both your weight loss goals and overall well-being.

Tailoring Exercise for Aging Bodies

Tailoring exercise for aging bodies is a key aspect of achieving fitness goals and promoting overall well-being. As our bodies age, they undergo changes in muscle mass, bone density, and flexibility. Here's a guide on how to customize your exercise routine for optimal results:

Strength Training:
- Prioritize resistance or strength training to maintain and build muscle mass.
- Incorporate weight-bearing exercises like squats, lunges, and resistance training with bands or weights.

Cardiovascular Exercise:

- Choose low-impact cardio activities like brisk walking, cycling, swimming, or elliptical training to protect joints.
- Aim for at least 150 minutes of moderate-intensity aerobic exercise per week.

Flexibility and Stretching:

- Include regular stretching exercises to improve flexibility and prevent stiffness.
- Practices like yoga or tai chi can be beneficial for balance and flexibility.

Balance Exercises:

- Integrate balance exercises to reduce the risk of falls.
- Simple activities like standing on one leg or incorporating balance-focused

movements into your routine can be effective.

Adapted Workouts:

- Be open to modifying exercises based on individual needs and limitations.
- Consult with a fitness professional or physical therapist for personalized guidance.

Rest and Recovery:

- Allow for adequate rest days to prevent overexertion and promote recovery.
- Listen to your body and adjust the intensity and frequency of workouts accordingly.

Mind-Body Connection:

- Incorporate mindfulness practices into your routine, such as meditation or deep breathing exercises.

These practices can enhance overall well-being and contribute to a positive mindset.

By tailoring your exercise routine to accommodate the changes that come with aging, you not only enhance physical fitness but also support joint health, balance, and mental well-being. Remember, the goal is to create a sustainable and enjoyable exercise regimen that aligns with your body's current needs and capabilities.

Hormonal Factors in Weight Gain

Understanding the impact of hormonal factors on weight gain is crucial, especially as our bodies undergo changes with age. Here are key hormonal factors that can contribute to weight gain:

Estrogen and Menopause (Women):
- A decline in estrogen during menopause can lead to an increase in abdominal fat.
- Hormonal shifts may also affect metabolism, making weight management more challenging.

Testosterone Decline (Men):
- With age, men experience a gradual decline in testosterone levels, which

can contribute to a decrease in muscle mass and an increase in body fat.

Insulin Sensitivity:

- Insulin resistance may increase with age, affecting the body's ability to regulate blood sugar.
- Poor insulin sensitivity can lead to weight gain, especially around the abdominal area.

Cortisol and Stress:

- Chronic stress can lead to elevated cortisol levels, promoting fat storage, particularly in the abdominal region.
- Managing stress through relaxation techniques is essential for hormonal balance.

Thyroid Function:

- Thyroid hormones play a role in metabolism, and imbalances can lead to weight fluctuations.
- Hypothyroidism (underactive thyroid) can contribute to weight gain.

Leptin and Ghrelin:

- These hormones regulate hunger and satiety.
- Imbalances can lead to increased appetite and difficulty in recognizing when you're full.

Understanding these hormonal influences is the first step in addressing weight gain.

Tailoring lifestyle choices, such as a balanced diet, regular exercise, stress management, and sufficient sleep, can help mitigate the impact of hormonal changes and support weight management goals. If concerns persist, consulting with a healthcare professional is advisable for a more personalized approach.

Strategies for Sustainable Weight Loss

Sustainable weight loss involves adopting strategies that are not only effective but also maintainable in the long term. Here are key strategies to support lasting success:

Realistic Goal Setting:
- Set achievable, realistic weight loss goals to avoid frustration and disappointment.
- Celebrate small milestones along the way.

Balanced Nutrition:
- Adopt a balanced and nutrient-dense diet that includes a variety of foods.
- Focus on portion control and mindful eating.

Regular Physical Activity:

- Engage in regular exercise that includes both cardiovascular activities and strength training.
- Find activities you enjoy to make exercise a sustainable part of your routine.

Lifestyle Modifications:

- Make sustainable lifestyle changes rather than opting for short-term, restrictive diets.
- Identify and address habits that may contribute to weight gain.

Mindful Eating:

- Pay attention to hunger and fullness cues.
- Avoid distractions while eating to promote awareness of food intake.

Adequate Sleep:

- Ensure you get sufficient, quality sleep as inadequate sleep can affect hunger hormones and metabolism.

Stress Management:

- Implement stress-reducing practices such as meditation, deep breathing, or yoga.
- Chronic stress can contribute to weight gain.

Hydration:

- Stay well-hydrated as dehydration can sometimes be mistaken for hunger.
- Choose water or other low-calorie beverages over sugary drinks.

Social Support:

- Seek support from friends, family, or a weight loss group.

- Having a support system can provide motivation and encouragement.

Behavioral Changes:

- Address emotional eating and identify triggers for unhealthy habits.
- Consider working with a behavioral therapist if needed.

Remember, sustainable weight loss is a gradual process. By focusing on lifestyle changes that you can realistically maintain, you increase the likelihood of not only losing weight but also keeping it off in the long run. Consult with healthcare or fitness professionals for personalized guidance based on your individual needs and health status.

Meal Planning Tips

Effective meal planning is a cornerstone of successful weight management. Here are practical meal planning tips to support your journey:

Plan Ahead:

- Take time to plan your meals for the week in advance.
- Create a shopping list based on your planned meals to avoid impulse purchases.

Balanced Plate:

- Aim for a balanced plate with a mix of lean proteins, whole grains, fruits, and vegetables.
- Include a variety of colors and textures for a diverse nutrient intake.

Portion Control:

- Be mindful of portion sizes to avoid overeating.
- Use smaller plates to create a visual cue for appropriate portions.

Prep Ingredients:

- Wash, chop, and prepare ingredients ahead of time for quick and convenient meals.
- Consider batch cooking for efficiency.

Include Snacks:

- Plan for nutritious snacks to curb hunger between meals.
- Opt for snacks that combine protein and fiber for sustained energy.

Hydration:

- Incorporate water or herbal teas into your meal plan.

- Sometimes, thirst can be mistaken for hunger.

Variety is Key:

- Experiment with different recipes and cuisines to keep meals interesting.
- Rotate your protein sources and try new vegetables to enhance nutritional diversity.

Mindful Eating:

- Sit down and savor your meals without distractions.
- Pay attention to hunger and fullness cues.

Flexibility:

- Allow flexibility in your meal plan to accommodate changes in schedule or unexpected events.
- Have a list of quick and healthy go-to options for busy days.

Incorporate Treats:

- Allow yourself occasional treats to satisfy cravings and prevent feelings of deprivation.
- Focus on moderation rather than strict restriction.

By incorporating these meal planning tips, you can create a sustainable and enjoyable approach to nourishing your body. Remember, meal planning is a tool to empower your choices, providing structure while allowing for flexibility in your journey toward healthier eating habits.

Effective Workouts for Adults over 40

For adults over 40, effective workouts should prioritize overall health, mobility, and strength. Here are workout suggestions tailored to this demographic:

Cardiovascular Exercise:
- Engage in moderate-intensity cardio activities like brisk walking, cycling, or swimming.
- Aim for at least 150 minutes per week, breaking it into manageable sessions.

Strength Training:
- Incorporate resistance training to maintain and build muscle mass.

- Focus on compound exercises like squats, lunges, and chest presses using weights or resistance bands.

Flexibility and Mobility:

- Include dynamic stretches and flexibility exercises to enhance joint mobility.
- Practices like yoga or Pilates can improve flexibility and balance.

Low-Impact Options:

- Choose low-impact exercises to protect joints.
- Options include elliptical training, stationary biking, or water aerobics.

Interval Training:

- Incorporate interval training to boost metabolism.

- Alternating between periods of higher intensity and lower intensity can be effective.

Core Strengthening:
- Prioritize core exercises to support posture and prevent back pain.
- Planks, bird-dogs, and stability ball exercises are beneficial.

Balance Exercises:
- Include activities that improve balance, reducing the risk of falls.
- Stand on one leg, try heel-to-toe walking, or incorporate balance-focused movements.

Listen to Your Body:
- Be attentive to how your body responds to exercise.

- Modify intensity and duration based on individual fitness levels and any existing health conditions.

Consistency Over Intensity:

- Prioritize consistency in your workout routine over extreme intensity.
- Regular, moderate exercise is key to long-term health.

Recovery:

- Allow sufficient time for recovery between sessions, especially if engaging in strength training.
- Include activities like foam rolling or gentle stretching on rest days.

Remember to consult with a healthcare professional or fitness expert before starting a new exercise program, especially if you have any pre-existing health conditions.

Tailoring your workouts to your individual needs and capabilities is essential for a safe and effective fitness routine.

Adequate Sleep and Stress Management

Adequate sleep and effective stress management play pivotal roles in overall well-being, especially when it comes to weight management. Here's why they are crucial and how to incorporate them into your routine:

Adequate Sleep:

- Lack of sleep can disrupt hormonal balance, leading to increased hunger and cravings, especially for high-calorie foods.
- Strive for 7-9 hours of quality sleep per night.
- Maintain a consistent sleep schedule, create a relaxing bedtime routine, and

ensure your sleep environment is conducive to rest.

Stress Management:

- Chronic stress triggers the release of cortisol, which can contribute to abdominal fat accumulation.

- Incorporate stress-reducing practices into your daily life, such as meditation, deep breathing exercises, or yoga.

- Identify stressors and work on strategies to address or cope with them effectively.

Mindfulness and Relaxation:

- Practice mindfulness to stay present and reduce anxiety about the past or future.

- Engage in activities that bring joy and relaxation, whether it's reading, listening to music, or spending time in nature.

Regular Physical Activity:

- Exercise is a powerful stress reducer and can improve sleep quality.
- Aim for a mix of cardiovascular activities, strength training, and flexibility exercises in your routine.

Establish Boundaries:

- Learn to say no and set healthy boundaries to prevent overwhelm.
- Prioritize self-care and allocate time for activities that bring joy and relaxation.

Quality Nutrition:

- Eat a balanced diet with nutrient-dense foods to support overall health, including foods rich in vitamins and minerals that aid stress management.

Hydration:

- Stay well-hydrated as dehydration can amplify the physical effects of stress.
- Limit caffeine intake, especially in the evening, to promote better sleep.

Disconnect from Screens:

- Limit screen time before bedtime to improve sleep quality.
- Blue light emitted by screens can interfere with the production of the sleep hormone melatonin.

By prioritizing adequate sleep and implementing effective stress management techniques, you create a foundation for not only weight management but also enhanced overall health and vitality. These practices contribute to a positive cycle, where improved sleep and stress management support your fitness and nutrition goals, and vice versa.

Hydration and Its Impact on Weight Loss

Hydration is a fundamental aspect of overall health and can significantly impact weight loss. Here's how staying well-hydrated plays a role in your weight management journey:

Appetite Regulation:

- Drinking water before meals can help control appetite, leading to reduced calorie intake.
- Sometimes, feelings of thirst can be confused with hunger, and staying hydrated can prevent unnecessary snacking.

Metabolism Boost:

- Adequate hydration supports metabolic processes, assisting in the efficient breakdown of nutrients.
- Water is essential for the proper function of enzymes involved in metabolism.

Calorie-Free Beverage Option:

- Choosing water as your primary beverage helps avoid the empty calories found in sugary drinks.
- Regular consumption of high-calorie beverages can contribute to weight gain.

Fluid Balance and Exercise Performance:

- Proper hydration is crucial for optimal exercise performance.

- Staying hydrated supports endurance, allowing you to engage in more effective workouts for weight loss.

Thermogenic Effect:
- Drinking cold water can slightly increase calorie expenditure as the body works to warm the water to body temperature.
- While the effect is modest, every little bit contributes to overall energy expenditure.

Reduced Water Retention:
- Paradoxically, staying well-hydrated can help prevent water retention.
- When the body is consistently hydrated, it's less likely to retain water, reducing bloating and the appearance of excess weight.

Hydration for Fat Metabolism:

- Proper hydration supports the body's ability to metabolize stored fat for energy.
- Inadequate water intake may hinder this process.

Satiety Signals:

- Dehydration can sometimes be misinterpreted by the body as a need for more food.
- Staying hydrated ensures clear signals between thirst and hunger.

To optimize hydration for weight loss, aim to drink an adequate amount of water throughout the day. Individual needs vary, but a common guideline is to consume at least 8 glasses (64 ounces) of water daily. Adjust this based on factors like climate, activity level, and individual health considerations. Integrating hydration into your overall wellness routine can positively impact your weight loss efforts and contribute to improved overall health.

Common Challenges and Solutions

Navigating weight loss, especially after 40, comes with its share of challenges. Here are some common hurdles and practical solutions:

Metabolism Slowdown:

- Challenge: Metabolism tends to slow down with age.
- Solution: Counteract this by incorporating regular strength training to maintain and build muscle mass, which can boost metabolism.

Hormonal Changes:

- Challenge: Hormonal shifts, especially in menopause or andropause, can contribute to weight gain.

- Solution: Focus on a balanced diet, exercise regularly, and consult with healthcare professionals for hormone-related guidance.

Busy Lifestyle:

- Challenge: Juggling work, family, and other responsibilities can make prioritizing health challenging.
- Solution: Plan and prepare meals in advance, schedule workouts as non-negotiable appointments, and incorporate quick, effective exercises into your routine.

Emotional Eating:

- Challenge: Using food as a coping mechanism for stress or emotions.
- Solution: Identify triggers for emotional eating, develop alternative coping strategies, and seek support

from friends, family, or a mental health professional.

Plateaus:

- Challenge: Weight loss progress may plateau.
- Solution: Adjust your workout routine, reassess your calorie intake, and consider incorporating new foods or activities to break through plateaus.

Inconsistent Sleep:

- Challenge: Poor sleep quality or insufficient sleep can impact weight loss efforts.
- Solution: Prioritize sleep hygiene, create a consistent sleep schedule, and address any underlying sleep issues.

Social Pressures:

- Challenge: Social events may involve tempting, calorie-dense foods.

- Solution: Plan ahead for social occasions, make healthier choices when possible, and practice moderation.

Lack of Support:

- Challenge: Feeling isolated in your weight loss journey.
- Solution: Seek support from friends, family, or join a weight loss group. Consider working with a nutritionist or personal trainer for professional guidance.

Unrealistic Expectations:

- Challenge: Expecting rapid or extreme results.
- Solution: Set realistic, achievable goals, celebrate small victories, and understand that sustainable weight loss takes time.

Medical Conditions:

- Challenge: Certain medical conditions can impact weight loss.
- Solution: Consult with healthcare professionals to address any underlying health issues and develop a weight loss plan tailored to your individual needs.

Each weight loss journey is unique, and it's normal to encounter challenges along the way.

By proactively addressing these challenges with practical solutions and maintaining a flexible, positive mindset, you can enhance your chances of long-term success.

Celebrating Small Victories

Celebrating small victories is an essential part of maintaining motivation and fostering a positive mindset on your weight loss journey. Here are ways to acknowledge and celebrate your achievements, no matter how small:

Set Milestones:

- Break your overall goal into smaller, achievable milestones.
- Celebrate reaching each milestone as a significant accomplishment.

Positive Self-Talk:

- Practice positive self-talk to acknowledge your efforts and progress.

- Replace self-criticism with self-encouragement.

Non-Scale Wins:

- Celebrate non-scale victories, such as improved energy levels, better sleep, or increased strength.
- These victories reflect positive changes in your overall well-being.

Reward System:

- Establish a reward system for reaching milestones.
- Choose rewards that align with your healthy lifestyle, such as a new workout gear or a relaxing spa day.

Share Achievements:

- Share your successes with friends, family, or a supportive community.
- Their encouragement can reinforce your sense of accomplishment.

Gratitude Journal:

- Keep a gratitude journal to reflect on the positive aspects of your journey.

- Express gratitude for the changes you've made and the progress you've achieved.

Reflect on Challenges Overcome:

- Acknowledge and celebrate the challenges you've overcome.

- Recognize your resilience and determination.

Take Progress Photos:

- Document your journey with progress photos.

- Seeing visible changes can be a powerful motivator and cause for celebration.

Healthy Treats:

- Treat yourself to small, healthy rewards.
- Enjoy a favorite healthy meal, indulge in a piece of dark chocolate, or take a leisurely walk in a scenic place.

Self-Care Rituals:

- Incorporate self-care rituals into your routine.
- Whether it's a relaxing bath, a massage, or a quiet moment with a good book, prioritize self-care as a celebration of your efforts.

By acknowledging and celebrating small victories, you cultivate a positive mindset that fuels your motivation for the long run. Remember, each step forward, no matter how small, contributes to your overall success. Celebrate your journey, embrace the progress you've made, and look forward to the continued achievements along the way.

Seeking Professional Guidance

Seeking professional guidance is a wise and proactive step on your weight loss journey, especially after 40. Here's why and how to go about it:

Individualized Approach:

- Why: Professionals, such as nutritionists, dietitians, or personal trainers, can provide personalized guidance based on your unique needs, preferences, and health status.
- How: Schedule consultations with these experts to discuss your goals, challenges, and receive tailored advice.

Health Assessment:

- Why: Healthcare professionals can conduct a thorough health assessment, considering factors like existing medical conditions, medications, and potential obstacles to weight loss.
- How: Consult with your primary care physician or a registered dietitian who can evaluate your health and provide recommendations.

Nutritional Guidance:

- Why: Nutritionists or dietitians can help design a balanced and sustainable meal plan that aligns with your weight loss goals.
- How: Seek the expertise of a registered dietitian who can offer evidence-based nutritional guidance.

Fitness Expertise:

- Why: Personal trainers or fitness professionals can create a workout plan tailored to your fitness level, preferences, and any physical limitations.

- How: Consider hiring a certified personal trainer for a few sessions to get started with a customized exercise routine.

Behavioral Support:

- Why: Behavioral therapists or psychologists can assist in addressing emotional eating, stress management, and behavior modification.

- How: Explore counseling services or work with a therapist who specializes in behavior change and emotional well-being.

Medical Supervision:

- Why: Individuals with certain health conditions may benefit from medical supervision during weight loss.
- How: Discuss your weight loss goals with your healthcare provider, who can offer guidance and monitor your progress.

Accountability and Motivation:

- Why: Having a professional provides accountability and motivation, crucial elements for long-term success.
- How: Regular check-ins, follow-up appointments, or training sessions with professionals can help you stay on track.

Educational Resources:

- Why: Professionals can provide educational resources and information to enhance your understanding of nutrition, exercise, and lifestyle factors.

- How: Attend workshops, seminars, or online courses offered by qualified experts in the field.

Remember, seeking professional guidance is an investment in your health and well-being. It enhances the effectiveness of your weight loss efforts and ensures that you receive evidence-based, individualized advice to support your journey. Whether you're focusing on nutrition, exercise, or behavioral changes, collaborating with professionals can significantly contribute to your success.

Conclusion

In conclusion, the journey of weight loss after 40 is a multifaceted exploration that goes beyond mere numbers on a scale. It is an empowering venture into understanding and adapting to the unique changes our bodies undergo with age. By embracing a holistic approach that encompasses balanced nutrition, tailored exercise, adequate sleep, stress management, and seeking professional guidance, you pave the way for sustainable and fulfilling transformation.

Recognizing the impact of hormonal factors, addressing metabolic shifts, and celebrating small victories become integral parts of this journey. The importance of hydration, thoughtful meal planning, and the incorporation of effective workouts for aging bodies further contribute to a comprehensive strategy for success.

Remember, each step forward, no matter how small, is a triumph worth celebrating. Whether it's the nourishment of your body through balanced meals, the invigoration of your muscles through purposeful exercise, or the restoration of your well-being through quality sleep and stress management – every choice matters.

In seeking professional guidance, you invest in a wealth of knowledge and support that propels you towards your goals. This journey is not about quick fixes; it's about creating sustainable habits and a positive relationship with your body that extends well beyond the initial weight loss.

So, embark on this transformative journey with confidence, patience, and a commitment to your well-being. The path may have its challenges, but each challenge is an opportunity to learn, grow, and ultimately thrive. Here's to a healthier, more vibrant you. Your journey continues, and the best is yet to come.

www.ingramcontent.com/pod-product-compliance
Lightning Source LLC
Chambersburg PA
CBHW050850260726
48660CB00006B/2541